Using Ginger

Planting, Culinary, Medical and Beauty Aspects

By
Gene Ashburner

ISBN-13:978-1502808684
ISBN-10:1502808684

Content

Ginger - Zingiber Officinale

Scientific Name

Zingiber Officinale Roscoe

Family

Zingiberaceae

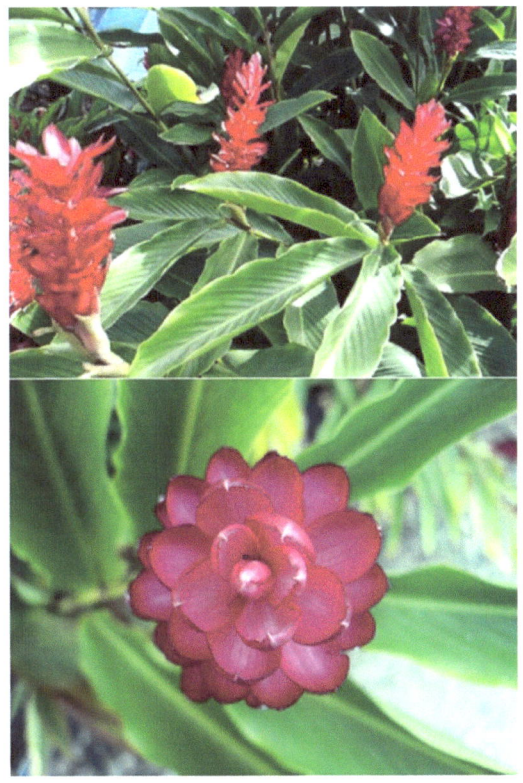

Ginger is one of the world's oldest and most important spices and is now widely grown. Other plants related to ginger are turmeric, cardamom, and galangal.

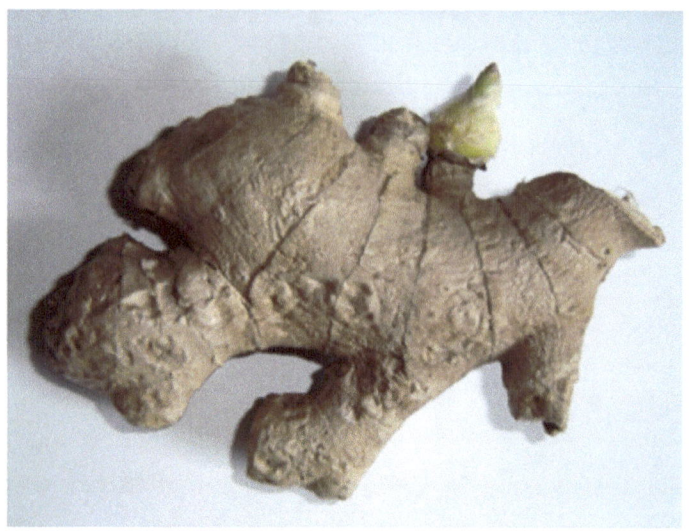

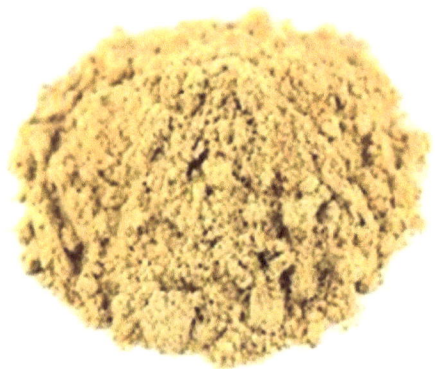

Fresh Ginger and Powdered Dry Ginger

How To Grow Ginger

Ginger is extremely easy to grow even indoors.

Step 1

Buy a smooth skinned, plump ginger rhizome (root) (don't get one that looks shrivelled as it will indicate an old root)

The fresh rhizome is knobbly, off-white or buff-coloured and often branched.

The pale yellow flesh should not be too fibrous.

Look for ginger rhizomes with well developed "eyes" or growth buds.

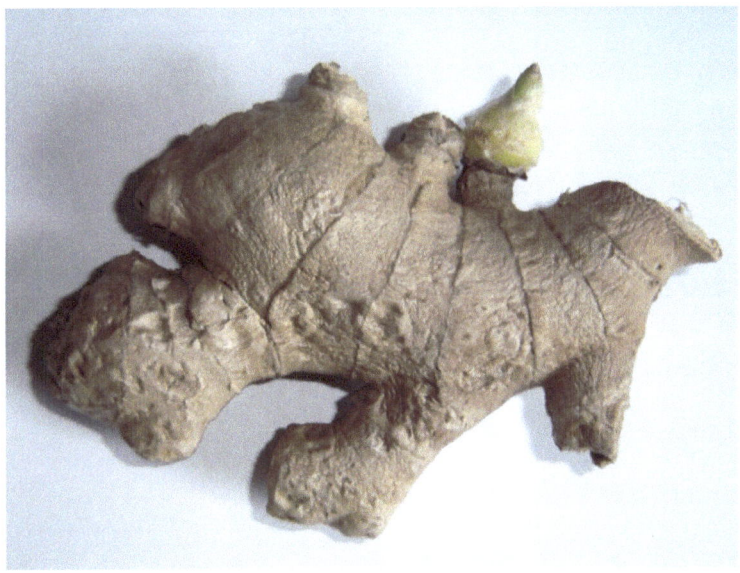

Step 2

Soak the ginger root in warm water overnight if it looks very dried out.

Step 3

Cut the soaked ginger root into smaller pieces allowing a few bumps per piece. You don't have to do this; a larger rhizome will also grow.

Step 4

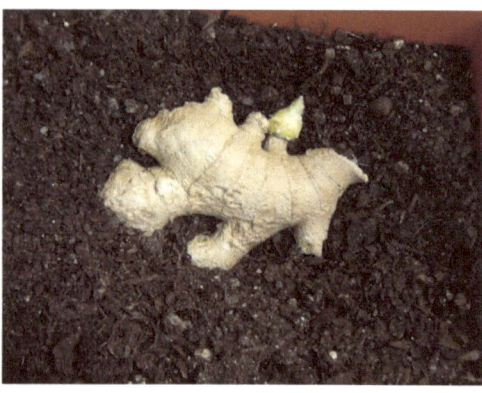

Fill a pot with good quality, moist and rich potting soil.

Make sure that the pot has good drainage.

Ginger needs rich and moist soil – not soggy soil!!

It does not need to be a huge pot as ginger plants don't take up much space and only grow 2 to 3 feet in height.

Step 5

Press the ginger root into the soil (not too deep - about 3 to 4 inches will be about right).

Cover the ginger root with soil.

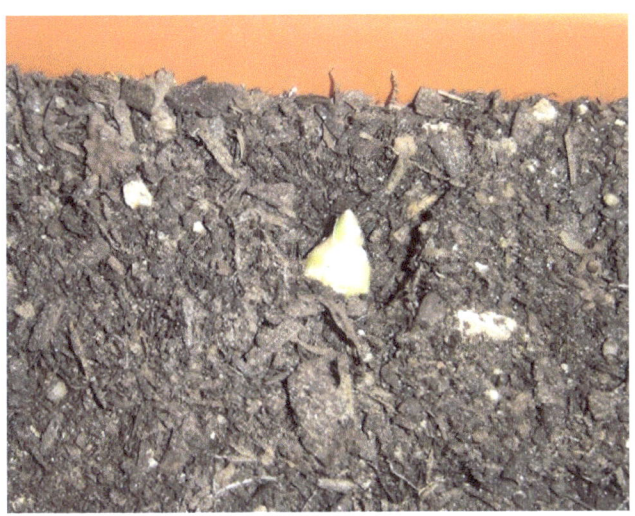

Step 6

Ginger likes a humid environment; so ensure that the ginger plant never dries out. Spraying the ginger plant with a spray bottle of water is a good idea, do this every other day.

Ginger also needs a sheltered, warm and partially sunny environment – at least 75 degrees.

Ginger does not like direct sun and wind.

How To Store Ginger

Ginger can be placed in a plastic bag and refrigerated or frozen.

Ginger – Different Options For Different Purposes

- Fresh green ginger
- Dried whole ginger
- Dried powdered ginger
- Candied ginger (see section – Candied Ginger for the recipe)
- Stem ginger or preserved ginger (see section – Stem Ginger / Preserved Ginger for the recipe)
- Ginger juice (see section – Ginger Juice for the recipe)
- Ginger tincture (see section – Ginger Tincture for the recipe)

Ginger Used For Culinary Purposes

Ginger has a hot slightly biting flavor. It is an essential ingredient in curries, pickles and many Asian vegetable dishes.

It is also used in gingerbread, biscuits, cakes, brownies, smoothies and puddings.

For baking purposes the ginger is mostly used in a dried, powdered form. Fresh ginger will be used for curries, candied ginger and pickles.

Fresh ginger and dried ginger are somewhat different in flavor.

Fresh ginger can be substituted for powdered ginger at a ratio of 6 to 1.

Fresh ginger may be peeled before using it for cooking or eating.

Candied Ginger

Candied ginger is the ginger root that has been cooked in sugar until soft. Candied ginger is then used as a type of confectionery or it is used in other baked confectionary.

Ingredients

1125 ml water

1125 ml sugar

375 ml ginger (sliced)

Additional sugar to coat the ginger

Method

Combine the sugar and water together in a saucepan.

Heat the mixture until the sugar has completely dissolved.

Bring the mixture to boiling point.

Reduce the heat.

Add the ginger pieces.

Boil the ginger mixture for 45 minutes.

Remove the ginger from the heat.

Place the ginger pieces onto a wire rack.

Leave the ginger pieces to dry for 30 minutes.

Toss the ginger pieces in the additional sugar to coat the ginger.

Place the ginger pieces on a parchment covered baking sheet.

Once the ginger pieces are dry, store them in an airtight container.

Stem Ginger / Preserved Ginger

Stem ginger or preserved ginger is young ginger that has been peeled and preserved in sugar syrup. The sugar syrup is sweet and will be used in sweet desserts and baking.

Ingredients

Young ginger (peeled and cut into small pieces)

Water to cover the ginger pieces in the saucepan (x3)

500 ml white sugar

750 ml soft brown sugar

750 ml water

Method

Place the ginger pieces in a saucepan.

Pour enough water in the saucepan to cover the ginger pieces.

Bring the water to boiling point.

Remove from the heat.

Strain the water off the ginger.

Place the ginger pieces back into the saucepan.

Repeat this process twice more i.e. the ginger pieces should be boiled 3 times.

Combine the brown sugar, white sugar and water together in another saucepan.

Bring the mixture to boiling point while dissolving the sugar.

Reduce the heat.

Simmer for 5 minutes.

Add the ginger pieces.

Boil for 30 minutes until the syrup has thickened.

Remove from the heat.

Cool the mixture completely.

Spoon the ginger pieces and syrup into sterilized jars.

Refrigerate the ginger before use.

Ginger Juice

Ingredients

Fresh ginger pieces

Method

Peel the ginger pieces.

Grate the peeled ginger.

Squeeze the juice out of the grated ginger.

Ginger Tincture

Ingredients

250 ml fresh ginger root (peeled)

500 ml Vodka

Method

Blend the fresh ginger root in a food processor.

Spoon the ginger root into a sterile glass jar.

Add the Vodka to the jar.

Seal the glass jar with a lid.

Leave the jar to stand for 2 weeks.

Shake the jar every day.

Strain the ginger mixture through a muslin cloth.

Pour the ginger liquid into a dark glass bottle.

Ginger Bread

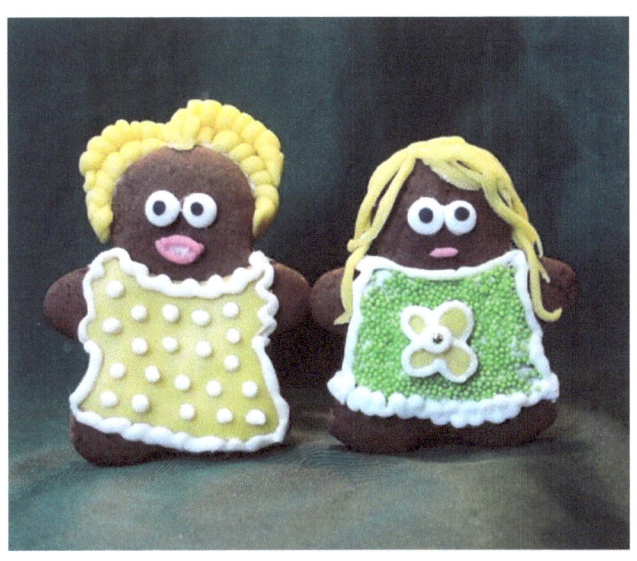

Gingerbread Recipe

Make Gingerbread Men And Gingerbread Houses

Ingredients

400 ml flour

10 ml powdered ginger

10 ml powdered cinnamon

5 ml salt

125 ml margarine

225 ml soft brown sugar

1 egg (beaten)

Method

Combine the flour, ginger, powdered cinnamon, and salt together.

Rub in the margarine.

Add the sugar.

Mix well.

Beat in the egg.

Mix well.

Cover the dough with plastic wrap.

Refrigerate to chill the dough.

Roll the gingerbread dough out onto a floured surface.

Use gingerbread men cutters to make gingerbread men and decorate as desired.

Use gingerbread house cutters to make a gingerbread house and decorate the gingerbread house as desired.

Ginger Banana Bread

Ingredients

250 ml butter

250 ml sugar

2 eggs (separated)

375 ml bananas (mashed)

12,5 ml lemon juice

1000 ml flour

25 ml custard powder

5 ml bicarbonate of soda

5 ml baking powder

5 ml powdered ginger

5 ml powdered cinnamon

2 ml salt

400 ml milk

Method

Beat the butter and sugar together until creamy.

Beat the egg yolks and add to the butter mixture.

Blend well.

Combine the bananas and the lemon juice together.

Add to the butter mixture.

Sift the flour, custard powder, bicarbonate of soda, baking powder, ginger, cinnamon and salt together.

Add the dry ingredients to the butter mixture.

Add the milk.

Whisk the egg whites until stiff.

Fold the egg whites into the butter mixture.

Pour the batter into a greased load pan.

Bake at 180 degrees C for about 45 minutes.

Ginger Cakes And Cookies

Powdered dry ginger is typically used as a flavoring for recipes such as gingerbread, cookies, cakes and puddings.

Ginger Apple Cup Cakes

Ingredients

  1000 ml diced apple

  500 ml sugar

  125 ml oil

  250 ml walnuts

  2 eggs

  5 ml powdered ginger

  250 ml flour

  10 ml baking soda

  5 ml salt

  125 ml shortening

  125 ml butter

  1000 ml icing sugar

  25 ml milk

  5 ml powdered ginger

  Apple slices tossed in lemon juice (to prevent oxidation)

Crystallized ginger (chopped)

Method

Combine the apples and sugar together.

Add the oil, walnuts, eggs, ginger, flour, baking soda and salt.

Mix well.

Place the cupcake cases onto a baking sheet.

Pour the batter into cupcake cases.

Bake at 180 degrees C for 15 minutes.

Remove the cupcakes from the oven.

Leave the cupcakes to cool on a wire rack.

Cream the shortening and butter until light and fluffy.

Gradually add the icing sugar, one cup at a time.

Blend well on medium speed.

Add the milk and beat until light and fluffy.

Add the ginger and mix well.

Place frosting in a piping bag.

Pipe the cupcakes with the frosting.

Decorate with apple slices and crystallized ginger.

Ginger Cookies

Ingredients

50 g margarine

60 g sugar

87,5 ml golden syrup

200 g flour

10 ml powdered ginger

Glace cherries

Method

Combine the margarine, sugar and syrup together in a saucepan.

Heat until the margarine has melted.

Add the flour and ginger.

Mix well.

Spoon the mixture onto a greased baking sheet.

Decorate each biscuit with a glace cherry.

Bake at 180 degrees C for 10 to 15 minutes.

Ginger Apricot Brownies

Ingredients

140 g butter (melted and cooled)

4 large eggs

350 g castor sugar

200 g flour

50 g crystallized ginger (chopped)

100 g walnuts (chopped)

50 g dried apricots (chopped)

5 ml powdered cinnamon

Method

Beat the eggs and sugar until light and creamy.

Add the melted butter.

Sift the flour and cinnamon together.

Combine the egg mixture and the flour mixture together.

Fold in the ginger, walnuts and apricot pieces.

Pour into a greased, square baking pan.

Bake at 170 degrees C for 30 to 35 minutes.

Be careful not to over bake, the mixture should be gooey on the inside.

Allow the cake to cool for a few minutes.

Remove from the pan and cool on a wire rack until completely cool.

Cut into squares.

Ginger Cream Tart

Ingredients

250 ml golden syrup

250 ml boiling water

2 ml powdered ginger

50 ml ginger preserve (chopped up)

30 ml corn flour

15 ml custard powder

200 g ginger cookies (crushed)

75 ml butter (melted)

Whipped cream for garnishing

Chocolate (grated for garnishing)

Method

Combine the cookies and the butter together.

Press into a greased tart dish.

Chill until needed.

Heat the syrup, water and the powdered ginger to boiling point.

Add the ginger preserve.

Combine the corn flour and custard powder with a little cold water and mix to make a paste.

Add to the syrup mixture and cook for 3 minutes, stirring continuously.

Pour the filling into the tart crust.

Allow the tart to cool.

Sprinkle the grated chocolate over the top.

Garnish with whipped cream.

Ginger Candy

These candy recipes make use of candied ginger pieces. Either make your own candied ginger (see recipe in book or buy store bought candied ginger).

Ginger Fruit Squares

Ingredients

500 ml mixed fruit (mixed peel, raisins and chopped candied ginger)

3 tablespoons brandy

3 tablespoons lemon juice

250 g margarine

125 ml sugar

1 tin condensed milk

2 packets cookies (crushed)

Method

Mix the fruit, brandy and lemon juice together.

Melt the margarine.

Add the sugar and condensed milk to the margarine.

Stir in the cookies.

Add the fruit mixture.

Press into a greased cake pan.

Allow to cool and set.

Cut into squares.

Ginger Jellies

Ingredients

20 g gelatin

100 ml cold water

400 g sugar

50 ml hot water

15 ml lemon juice

100 g candied ginger (chopped)

50 g corn flour

50 g icing sugar

Method

Soak gelatin in cold water

Dissolve sugar in hot water and boil for 10 minutes.

Add gelatin to sugar water and boil for 15 minutes.

Add lemon juice and ginger.

Allow the mixture to cool.

Pour into dampened cake pan and cut into squares.

Allow the jellies to set for 2 hours.

Mix the icing sugar and corn flour together.

Remove from pan and dust with corn flour and icing sugar mixture.

Ginger Desserts

Powdered dry ginger is typically used as a flavoring for recipes such cakes and puddings.

Boiled Ginger Pudding

Ingredients

1,25 liter water

500 ml sugar

500 ml flour

10 ml powdered cinnamon

5 ml powdered ginger

2 ml salt

200 ml milk

10 ml bicarbonate of soda

25 ml apricot jam

30 ml butter

Method

Heat the water and sugar in a saucepan to boiling point.

Combine flour, cinnamon, ginger and salt together.

Mix the bicarbonate of soda into the milk.

Rub the butter and jam into the flour mixture.

Add the milk to the flour mixture.

Mix well.

Turn the heat down.

Spoon the batter into the boiling syrup.

Place a lid onto the saucepan and cook for 25 minutes without lifting the lid.

Serve warm.

Ginger Ice Cream

Stem ginger is sometimes called preserved ginger. It is young ginger roots that have been peeled and preserved in sugar syrup.

Ingredients

1 tin condensed milk

1 tin evaporated milk (chilled)

4 pieces stem ginger (chopped into cubes)

2 tablespoons ginger syrup from the stem ginger jar

Method

Beat the evaporated milk then add the condensed milk.

Add the pieces of stem ginger and ginger syrup.

Mix thoroughly.

Pour into a freezer-proof bowl and freeze for 6 hours.

Stir occasionally until mixture has frozen.

Ginger Drinks

Ginger works well in smoothies as it is a great digestive aid.

Ginger Apple Smoothie

Ingredients

2 granny Smith apples (peeled, cored and chopped)

2 lemons (peeled, pips removed and chopped)

250 ml water

250 ml ice

1 piece fresh ginger root (peeled and chopped)

Method

Combine all the ingredients together in a blender.

Blend until smooth.

Drink immediately.

Ginger Beer

Ingredients

4,5 litres cold water

750 ml sugar

25 g active dry yeast

30 ml ginger powder

5 ml cream of tartar

125 ml seeded raisins (bruise the raisins)

Method

Mix the sugar, water, yeast, ginger, cream of tartar and raisins (bruised) together.

Cover and let beer stand for 24 hours at room temperature.

Pour through a muslin cloth and pour into bottles.

Chill before serving.

Ginger Coconut Smoothie

Ingredients

62,5 ml apple juice

37,5 ml virgin coconut oil

½ banana (peeled and sliced)

2 ml fresh ginger root (peeled and grated)

125 ml coconut milk

Method

Combine all the ingredients together in a blender.

Blend until smooth.

Serve immediately.

Ginger Tea

Ingredients

Few slices fresh ginger root or 5 ml powdered ginger

250 ml boiling water

5 ml honey (optional)

Sliced orange or lemon (optional to add flavor)

Method

Combine the ginger and boiling water together.

If you are using fresh ginger, steep the ginger slices in the boiling water for at least 5 minutes.

Strain the ginger tea.

Add honey if desired.

Add orange or lemon slices if so desired – adds to the ginger tea taste.

Drink the ginger tea hot or cold

Ginger Used For Medicinal Purposes

Ginger is extremely versatile and can be taken as a tea, in crystallized form, dried and powdered form or as a tincture.

Ginger is also available in capsule form.

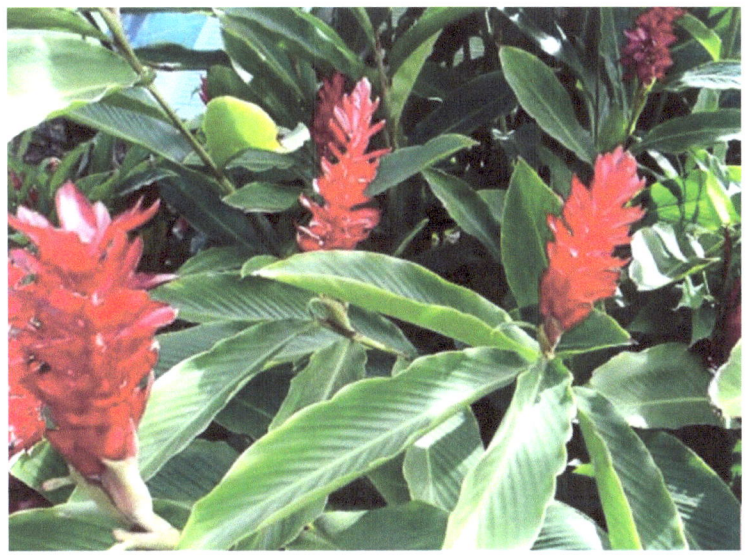

Acid Reflux And Digestive Remedy

Ginger can be used as a home remedy for acid reflux. Ginger is widely used as a digestive aid.

Ginger is also a natural remedy used to relieve heartburn.

Ingredients

Few slices fresh ginger root or 5 ml powdered ginger

250 ml boiling water

5 ml honey (optional)

Method

Combine the ginger and boiling water together.

If you are using fresh ginger, steep the ginger slices in the boiling water for at least 5 minutes.

Strain the ginger tea.

Add honey if desired.

Drink the ginger mixture after each meal.

Do this 3 times per day.

Circulation And Thinning Blood Remedy

Ginger is used to thin the blood and improve circulation. Ginger is one of the best defences against poor blood circulation.

Ginger tincture is easily absorbed by the body which helps in reducing the cholesterol level, cleansing the blood, preventing heart disease and also fights atherosclerosis.

Ginger Tea Remedy:

Ingredients

Few slices fresh ginger root or 5 ml powdered ginger

250 ml boiling water

5 ml honey (optional)

Method

Combine the ginger and boiling water together.

If you are using fresh ginger, steep the ginger slices in the boiling water for at least 5 minutes.

Stain the ginger tea.

Add honey if desired.

Drink at least 3 cups of this ginger tea per day.

Ginger Tincture Remedy:

Ingredients

20 drops ginger tincture

Water

Method

Dilute the ginger tincture in water.

Drink the ginger tincture mixture once per day.

Coughs And Colds Remedy

Ginger is used as a remedy for coughs and colds. Tea brewed from ginger is a common folk remedy used for preventing colds.

Ginger Tea For Colds:

Ingredients

Few slices fresh ginger root or 5 ml powdered ginger

250 ml boiling water

5 ml honey (optional)

Method

Combine the ginger and boiling water together.

If you are using fresh ginger, steep the ginger slices in the boiling water for at least 5 minutes.

Stain the ginger tea.

Add honey if desired.

Drink at least 3 cups of this ginger tea per day.

Cough Syrup Recipe:

Ingredients

250 ml water

250 ml honey

50 ml powdered ginger

Method

Combine the water, honey and ginger together in a saucepan.

Bring to the boil.

Reduce the heat.

Simmer the mixture until the mixture has reduced by half.

Remove from the heat.

Leave the mixture to cool.

Strain the liquid.

Pour the strained liquid into a container.

Store the cough syrup in the refrigerator.

Headaches Remedy

Ginger relieves and prevents headaches.

It is an anti-inflammatory and also has substances that help to reduce pain.

Ingredients

Few slices fresh ginger root or 5 ml powdered ginger

250 ml boiling water

5 ml honey (optional)

Method

Combine the ginger and boiling water together.

If you are using fresh ginger, steep the ginger slices in the boiling water for at least 5 minutes.

Stain the ginger tea.

Add honey if desired.

Drink the ginger tea.

Haemorrhoids Remedy

Ginger root has been used for centuries for digestive problems. Ginger root also contains antioxidant and anti-microbial properties and these properties will help hemorrhoids shrink

For Internal Hemorrhoids:

Ingredients

Ginger root (cut into small pieces - approximately 5 cm in length)

Method

Use the ginger root pieces as a suppository.

Continue using the ginger root suppositories for 7 days.

For External Hemorrhoids:

Ingredients

5 ml ginger powder

Balsam oil

Method

Combine the ginger powder and just enough Balsam oil together to form a paste.

Mix well.

Place the paste onto the affected area.

Cover the paste with a protective film.

Leave overnight.

Wash the mixture off the next morning.

Repeat the procedure for 7 days.

Inflammation And Infection Remedy

Ginger root contains properties that will alleviate inflammation and infection.

Drink the following concoction daily.

Ginger Tea Concoction Recipe

Ingredients

Few slices fresh ginger root or 5 ml powdered ginger

250 ml boiling water

5 ml honey (optional)

Method

Combine the ginger and boiling water together.

If you are using fresh ginger, steep the ginger slices in the boiling water for at least 5 minutes.

Stain the ginger tea.

Add honey if desired.

Drink at least 3 cups of this ginger tea per day.

Menstruation Relief Remedy

Ginger can be used as a pain relief remedy during menstruation.

Ingredients

5 ml powdered ginger

250 ml boiling water

5 ml honey (optional)

Method

Combine the ginger and boiling water together.

If you are using fresh ginger, steep the ginger slices in the boiling water for at least 5 minutes.

Stain the ginger tea.

Add honey if desired.

Drink the mixture all at once.

Nausea, Motion Sickness And Morning Sickness Remedy

Ginger is used to prevent nausea, motion sickness and morning sickness.

Powdered Ginger Remedy:

Ingredients

5 ml powdered ginger

250 ml boiling water

5 ml honey (optional)

Method

Combine the ginger and boiling water together.

If you are using fresh ginger, steep the ginger slices in the boiling water for at least 5 minutes.

Stain the ginger tea.

Add honey if desired.

Drink the ginger mixture once per day.

Ginger Tincture Remedy:

Ingredients

20 drops ginger tincture

Water

Method

Dilute the ginger tincture in water.

Drink the ginger tincture mixture once per day.

Candied Ginger Remedy:

Candied ginger is an effective remedy for motion sickness.

Sore Throat Remedy

Ingredients

Small piece of fresh ginger (peeled)

Method

Use the fresh ginger as a throat lozenge.

Ginger Used For Beauty Purposes

Acne Remedy

Ingredients

5 ml powdered ginger

50 ml milk

Cotton balls

Method

Combine the ginger and milk together.

Mix well.

Apply the ginger mixture onto the affected area with a cotton ball.

Ginger Rosemary Dandruff Treatment

Ingredients

37,5 ml olive oil

5 ml powdered ginger

5 ml rosemary oil

Method

Combine the olive oil, ginger and rosemary oil together

Mix well.

Massage the mixture into the scalp.

Leave for approximately 60 minutes.

Wash with shampoo and rinse hair.

Shiny Hair

If you want shiny hair then you need to eat ginger.

Ginger Used For Home Purposes

Ginger, Orange And Almond Air Freshener

Ingredients

750 ml water

3 oranges (sliced)

1 large piece of fresh ginger (sliced)

10 ml almond extract

Method

Combine the water, orange slices, ginger slices and almond extract together in a slow cooker or crock-pot.

Simmer the mixture on Low.

Keep adding water as the water evaporates.

The room will smell lovely.